# The Pain Free Office: How to Fix Your Desk and Your Posture

James Y. Marles

B.Sc, R. Kin

# Legal Disclaimer

**Warning**: All the information provided in The Pain-Free Office: How to Fix Your Desk and Your Posture is for educational and resource purposes only. It is not a substitute for or in addition to any advice given to you by your physician or health care provider.

Consult your physician before making any changes to your lifestyle. You are solely responsible for the way information in The Pain-Free Office: How to Fix Your Desk and Your Posture is perceived and used and so, you do so at your own risk.

In no way will James Marles or Informed Safety be held responsible for any injuries or problems that may occur due to the use of this guide or the advice contained within.

I would like to thank my family, friends, mentors, and teachers for their incredible support in writing this book and their continued guidance.

# Table of Contents

# Preface

This book has helped keep myself and my wife sane for the past year. I, much like most of the world, have been stuck inside under some form of quarantine for the better part of 2020 and 2021. At the beginning of 2020, the move to remote work was quite sudden due to the pandemic. The transition from having a "proper" computer workstation to a laptop and dining table office made me realize the challenges that I, and many other office workers encountered. Remote work, while beneficial in work flexibility and reduced commute, has forced many workers into poor and uncomfortable working conditions due to limited equipment to properly set up a home office.

Having spent most of my adult years learning and applying ergonomics, I had the knowledge and understanding to create a better setup for myself. However, this was not the case for many of my colleagues who do not have the same background. It was that realization which led me to writing this guide. I wanted to create an easy-to-follow but detailed book to help educate others to recognize and correct ergonomic hazards with the goal of preventing the build-up of pain and discomfort while working remotely and the subsequent return to the office.

It may sound crazy, but I absolutely loved the time and effort I put into this book. Condensing over 12 years of formal education, work experience, and trial-and-error was a great experience and I believe that you, the reader, will benefit from this guide. The book has been organized the mimic the flow of what I would cover while assessing a client at their office. As you work your way through, you will learn how small changes can make big differences in setting up a workstation and how those same changes can prevent or reduce discomfort from injuries such as "text neck, carpal tunnel syndrome, lower back pain, and many others.

The principles we will be going over in this guide will not be a "magic bullet" to heal or correct all ailments. They will, however, give you the foundations and knowledge to set up your workstation to fit YOU.

For extra ergonomic content, including free downloadable checklists, quick reference guides, and more, check out my website **www.informedsafety.com** and subscribe to our monthly newsletter where you'll get access to exclusive content, updates on upcoming events, and new content.

If you have any questions or would like to connect with me you can find all of my social links on my website.

# Introduction

To understand the goal of this guide, we need to start by defining what ergonomics is. The definition that I believe fits best is:

"The study of people and their interaction with the elements of their job or task including equipment, tools, facilities, processes, and environment."

With this definition in mind, the goal of this guide is to educate you on how you can adjust any computer workstation to better suit you.

There are various terms used to define ergonomic related injuries. These terms can include: Repetitive Strain Injuries (RSI), Cumulative Trauma Disorders (CTD), or Overuse Syndrome, to name a few. However, in this guide we will use the term "Musculoskeletal Disorders (MSD)" as it does not limit our view to only repetitive injuries. It is also important to understand that ergonomic injuries can be acute (caused by a single event) or they can be something developed over longer periods of time (cumulative/chronic), and they are rarely as a result of one specific task or job, but rather a combination of different issues.

Ergonomics and its principles can be used in several applications, not just in the office. To ensure the highest quality of information provided to you in this guide, we will focus on computer-based workstations and the principles applicable to a typical office.

To provide easy-to-reference material, this guide is broken down into six sections to focus on the different aspects of a workstation. The starting point will be an introduction to the basic concepts of ergonomics. This will get you thinking about and looking for the physical aspects of your office (posture, equipment, and movement). We will then go over the specific components that make up a typical workstation starting at the chair and finishing with peripherals (cellphone, documents, etc.). Each section will provide you with methods of minimizing discomfort and promoting healthy positioning, both through the introduction of new equipment or low/no-cost alternatives to achieve positive results.

This guide will not focus on having "perfect posture" or expensive equipment, though we will cover them in general within each section. The aim is to empower you to adjust your office specifically to your needs and comforts with what you have available.

Before we start, I would like to take a moment to talk about those of you who may be returning from a prolonged absence, such as medical or parental leave, and to provide some specific advice. For example, I took a parental leave from work to care for my newborn daughter so that my wife could go back to work earlier. I was fortunate to have had that opportunity and would encourage any new parent to do so. However, I had to make sure that when I returned to work, I increased my workload gradually. We need to understand that our bodies take time to adjust to changes, and after 6 months of changing diapers and napping on couches, I knew that sitting in an office would require some re-adjustment time. I would encourage everyone to discuss with your employer and medical practitioner ways to gradually increase your workload, or if there is a return-to-work process available. These simple actions can help you better transition back to an office environment and reduce the risk of developing discomfort.

Keep in mind that movement and variability throughout the day is still the best way to minimize discomfort, no matter how you decide to adjust your work space and what equipment or changes you make. I don't mean switching from a laptop to a cellphone, but more in terms of getting up and moving around or making "micro" adjustments to your setup. The change in your posture when you get up and walk around "resets" your awareness while also promoting blood flow to your muscles and tissues. When returning to a seated position, you are more likely to be aware of your posture and will go back to the "neutral" or ergonomic position that the workstation has been adjusted to promote.

With that said, let's take a look at your workspace and start making changes to get you happier and healthier.

# Section 1: Basic Concepts

Lack of awareness and education in the basic concepts of office ergonomics has been one of the largest hurdles for individuals looking to make ergonomic changes to their workstation. It is difficult for someone with no background in ergonomics to understand what an ergonomic hazard could be and how to identify and correct them. A great way to jump start your awareness, if possible, is to have a colleague or family member take a profile photo of you at your computer (a photo from the side) – it will give you a third-person perspective on how you sit at the computer and interact with the equipment. See *Fig. 2.1: The Chair* for an example.

Now that you have an idea of how you sit, we need to find and promote your "neutral" postures.

Upper body postures that we want to identify and avoid include: rounded back, hunched shoulders, head forwards, and bent wrists. These postures can have negative impacts on your health and can lead to injuries in the near future and long term if not addressed. The upper-body postures that we want to promote are: head above the shoulders (ears lined up with your shoulder), a "natural" curve in the spine, elbows relaxed at the sides (directly below the shoulders), and wrists that are flat and in line with the forearms. These postures aim to reduce pressure points at joints and decrease the constant muscle activation to maintain position.

For the lower body, we want to avoid sitting on one foot, tucking the feet underneath the chair, leaning to the left or right, sitting on unstable surfaces, and unsupported feet. We will focus on promoting having feet flat on the floor or on a raised surface, if necessary; knees bent at slightly greater than 90°; hips and lower back supported by the seat and backrest; and spacing between the front edge of the seat and the back of your knees.

When seated, you want to make sure you are using a comfortable and supportive chair – no hard surfaces, such as a wooden chair, or unsupportive, such as a bar stool or exercise ball (we will discuss the pros and cons of exercise balls in the next section). This will reduce contact pressure at the back, hips, and legs to promote blood circulation while allowing the muscles to relax and be supported by the chair.

When we talk about seated posture, traditional ergonomics has focused on specific angles or a "standard template" of how people should be sitting at the desk. While this may be beneficial in a controlled environment, it is poorly adapted for the real world. The more effective approach is to understand and utilize frequent adjustments depending on the task at hand and your comfort level. By doing this throughout the day, you can continuously cater the workstation to how you are feeling, optimizing it for you. To ensure you are equipped with the knowledge and skills to create the ideal workstation for you, we must understand that there are several individual differences that can change how we make adjustments. Differences such as footwear, eyewear, and height, to name a few, will be discussed in their respective sections.

# Section 2: The Chair

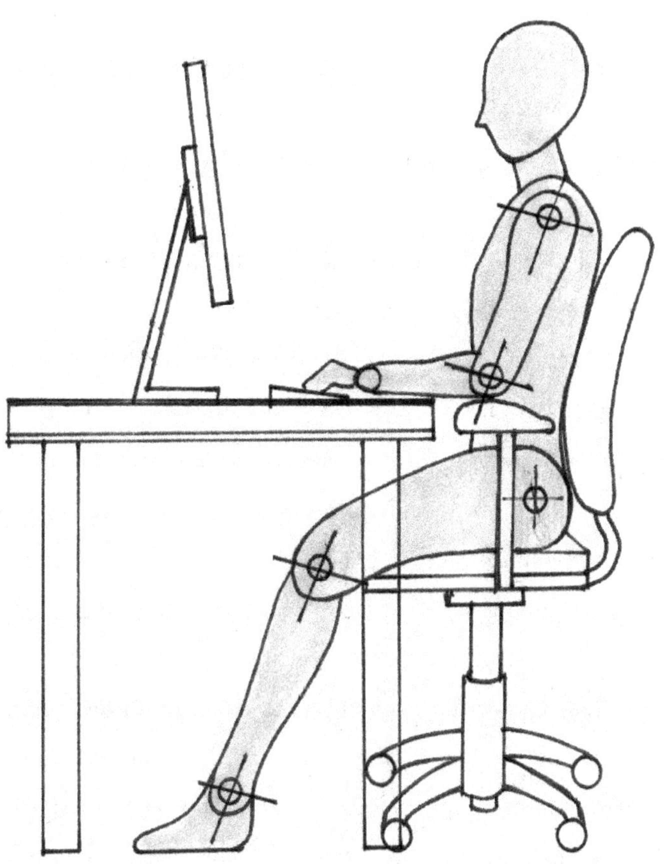

**Figure 2.1**: The Chair

## But First, Footwear

Before we look at adjusting your chair, let's discuss footwear as it will impact the adjustments made in this and later sections. Your choices in footwear will need to be considered when you are setting up your chair, depending on if you are working from home or in the office. If you are adjusting your workstation now, or have had an ergonomic assessment in the past, ask yourself, "Am I wearing the same shoes?" "Will I wear these shoes all the time?" Chances are the answer is "No". Some people change their shoes each day, others may change them depending on what they are doing, and some may prefer not to wear shoes while at the desk. I, for example, wear runners or dress shoes to work for personal comfort and, to some extent, fashion. However, I will change into safety boots if I am inspecting construction sites or working in industrial spaces. Footwear changes must be accounted for when you are setting up your chair as the heel height can affect your optimum seat height as well as foot support. It goes back to the point we mentioned earlier, of micro-adjustments to your workstation. Wearing a higher-heeled shoe requires a higher seat height, keyboard/mouse, and monitor(s). Wearing comfortable shoes at work that are not too tight and provide good foot and arch support can minimize the habit of tucking your feet under your chair or sitting on one foot.

Now that we have covered footwear, let's examine your chair. How you adjust your chair will affect your back posture, keyboard and mouse heights, monitor positioning, etc. There are basic adjustability features that you should look for in a chair, to provide you with the flexibility and adjustability to fit you. Features such as seat height, armrest height, and backrest angle adjustability are the three that I recommend as a minimum from an office chair that you will use for the majority of your day. Take a look underneath your current chair to see what handles and adjustments it has and try these out to give you an idea of what they can do and how much adjustability they provide. If you do not have access to a chair with these features, don't worry, we will go over some office "hacks" to provide you with the adjustability to make any chair fit you better.

I encourage you to consider the material that your chair is made of as this can play a large role in your comfort. While this will not be a topic in the guide, having a chair with breathable fabrics, such as cloth or mesh, is preferred over leather or wood. Cloth or mesh chairs allow the body to easily regulate temperature and can help reduce contact pressure from hard surfaces.

## Seat Pan

With your current footwear in mind, adjusting your chair starts with the seat height. You want your feet flat on the floor and knees at a 95° angle. This will provide support for the legs to decrease pressure on the hamstrings/thighs, and allow for proper circulation in the lower legs. If you switch shoes at work, you must adjust your chair to account for the change in heel height. You should also consider that if you are working on a surface higher than the elbows, and are unable to adjust surface height, it will lead to "shrugging" of the shoulders, a contributor to shoulder and neck tension. If using a chair that does not have height adjustability, such as a dining room chair, sit on a cushion to give you a boost. Don't forget to make sure you have support for your feet.

Once your seat height is adjusted, you want to make sure you have good spacing behind your knees to reduce pressure on the blood vessels. An easy way to measure this is by fitting 2-3 fingers between the front edge of the seat and the back of your knees. If you have to sit further forward to get this spacing, place a cushion between you and the backrest to maintain back support, or adjust the seat depth/backrest if possible.

Much like the seat depth, we should also consider the width of your seat. Typically, this is not an adjustable feature on a chair. The width of your hips is something that should be considered if you are able to change your chair or if you are looking to purchase a new one for your home office. Seat width should be slightly wider than the width of your hips to provide a stable support for the hips and legs. This will aid in reducing muscle use when seated, to prevent tightness from building up.

While we are on the subject of seats, I want to address the recent increase in the use of exercise balls as an alternative to traditional chairs. While these devices do promote users to use their core muscles to maintain posture, there is limited adjustability and no support for the upper body and lower back. I would strongly caution anyone using an exercise ball as a chair to treat it like an exercise device. Use it for short durations with plenty of rest in between, either by getting up and walking around, or by sitting in a more supportive chair. With prolonged use of an exercise ball, the muscles in the core, back, legs, and hips become fatigued. This can lead to slouching, muscle tightness, and discomfort in the lower back, which is the opposite of its purpose. There are some exercise balls that come with a base to provide more stability. However, it is still unable to fully address back support and you should change chairs or take a physical break when you begin to slouch or notice tightness or fatigue in the legs and hips.

## Footrests

Footrests can be introduced to supplement lower limb support if you are seated on a chair that is too high and it cannot be lowered. By placing a footrest underneath your feet, we can allow for the flexibility of sitting on higher chairs without causing increased pressure on the lower limb circulation. Ideally, the footrest is one that has both height and angle adjustability.

Some individuals may use a footrest to provide relief and posture variability in the lower limbs due to poor circulation or other health issues. By increasing the variety in lower limb positions throughout the day, we can promote circulation, reduce muscle tension and reduce muscle fatigue, thus improving lower limb health. If you are considering having a footrest at the desk, look for one with angle adjustability at a minimum and height adjustability if available. This will give you the added flexibility to adapt to changes in footwear.

## Backrest

Having an office chair with a comfortable backrest, where the top of the backrest reaches your shoulders, will give support to the upper body and back while seated. You can supplement any chair with a cushion or back support pad to add more adjustability. Adjusting your backrest to a slight recline (~100° angle), if you spend most of your time at the computer reading/writing emails or documents, or more upright at an angle of 90-95° for detailed work, will help support the upper body in a "neutral" position to reduce muscle and joint strain.

Once you have attained the desired angle, you will then adjust the height of your backrest to reach your shoulders. Chairs with shorter backrests do not provide enough support to the shoulders and upper back which can lead to hunched or "rounded" shoulders. Rounding of the spine is one of the contributing factors to developing neck and lower back discomfort as it leads to additional pressure on the spine, where the weight of the head and shoulders is no longer in line with the spine. A backrest that is too high or with a headrest that is too far forward, especially for individuals who have their hair tied back, can cause the head to be pushed forwards, leading to neck strain and discomfort.

Typically found within the backrest, and something you should never overlook, is the lumbar support. Some chairs may have a built-in adjustable system, but many do not, especially chairs in the lower price range. Purchasing a separate lumbar support to be used with your chair is a cost-effective alternative to provide the missing support, with the added bonus that it can be used in any chair, from the car to an airplane. Look for adjustable lumbar supports, such as inflatable ones, to customize the support in any seat without taking up much space in your bag.

External lumbar support should be placed in the small of your lower back to support the natural curvature of the spine. An easy method for locating the small of the back is, when standing, to slide your hand down along the spine from the ribs to where your back curves in the furthest, generally a finger or two above the hips. This inner curve to the spine is the lumbar region of your back and is typically where people experience their lower back pain. The support should be placed in the center of this curve and adjusted to support without pressing the back too far forward or allowing it to round out too much.

## Armrests

Once you are happy with the position of your backrest, let's move on to adjust the armrests to support the shoulders and upper back to prevent you from slouching or hunching. Office chairs can come with or without armrests, so depending on individual preference and arm length, you may or may not choose to use them.

For most people, armrests are beneficial when adjusted correctly. Having the armrest height set at or slightly above resting elbow height will support the shoulders and reduce neck and shoulder tension build-up from muscle use. The armrests should also be adjusted close to the body to prevent leaning more on one side, which can contribute to shoulder or hip discomfort.

Armrest depth will affect how close you sit to the desk or keyboard. If they are too far forward or too long, you may end up reaching when working. There are a few different ways to help with armrests that are too long. One method is to lower the armrests so that they fit under the desk or keyboard surface, but this is dependent on having adequate desk and keyboard surface space to support the forearms. Alternatively, some individuals may choose to remove the armrests completely and take more frequent rest and stretch breaks. This is not ideal for individuals who spend a large portion of their day typing as the shoulders lose out on their support. If you are unable to lower or remove your chair armrests, you can choose to sit further forward on the seat, keeping in mind to adjust your leg and backrest support, e.g., through the use of a backrest support pad. Note that not all chairs are built the same, e.g., some armrests may not provide a comfortable surface for the elbows to rest on. Armrests that are too firm can lead to pressure on the circulation and nerves in the elbow, causing issues down the forearms and into the wrists and hands. We want to ensure that the armrests have comfortable padding, either built into the chair, or purchased and installed separately. Reducing the pressure on the elbows is beneficial for those who have tendonitis, also known as golfer's or tennis elbow, as it reduces pressure at these locations.

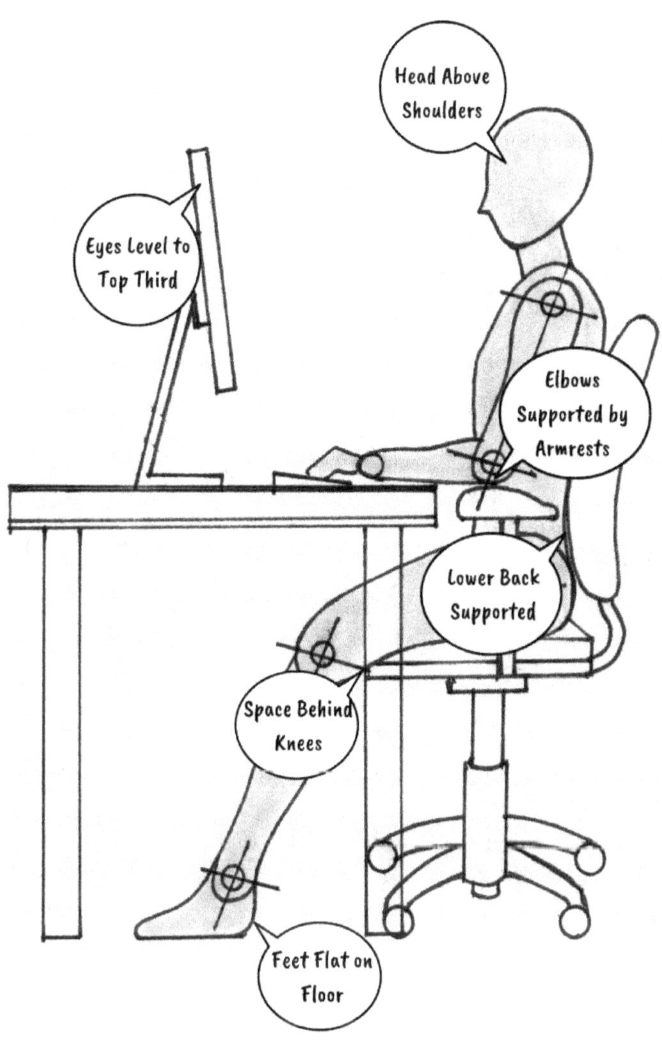


**Figure 2.2**: The Chair Quick Reference

# Section 3: Keyboard and Mouse

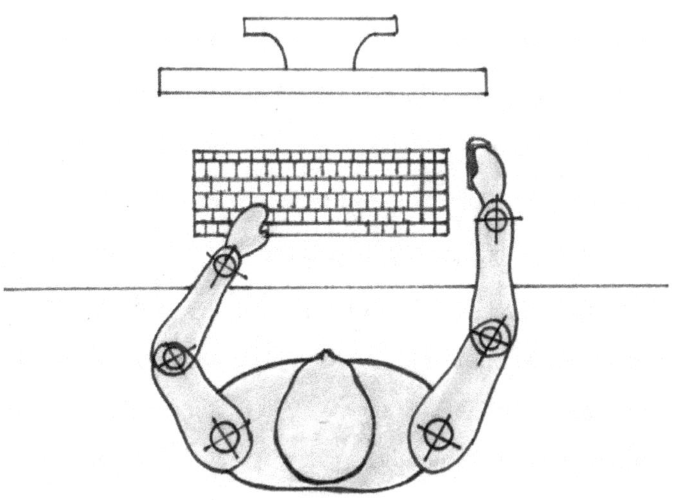

**Figure 3.1**: Keyboard and Mouse

With your chair set up and adjusted to your comfort, we will move on to the keyboard and mouse. These devices allow you to connect to your computer and can be a factor in determining hand and arm discomfort. By targeting the keyboard and mouse, where most of our time is spent at the computer, we can promote a healthier hand and wrist posture, reducing the risk of discomfort and injury.

## Keyboard Surface

Much like the height of your chair, the keyboard surface plays an integral role in positioning the body. Most of you working from home will have your keyboard and mouse set up on a "fixed" surface, such as a desk, dining table, or the kitchen counter. While these surfaces provide stability, they don't match up with how your chair is adjusted, and can lead to pressure points at the wrists and forearms. This can cause you to raise your shoulders in a "shrugged" position, which can lead to discomfort.

First, we will discuss how to adjust the keyboard and mouse height on a fixed surface. The easiest method is to adjust your seat height to match. If, for example, your keyboard is too high, raising the chair height to have your elbows, or armrests, level to the keyboard surface will provide a smooth transition between the chair support and the keyboard. This will allow the elbows and shoulders to stay relaxed while reducing pressure on the wrists and forearms.

If your keyboard and mouse surface are too low, this can lead to hunching of the shoulders and back, as well as creating more pressure on the wrists and forearms from leaning. Rather than working on a higher surface, you could lower your seat height. If seat height cannot be lowered, place something under the keyboard and mouse to raise it higher. Items such as an empty box or books that are the same height are great, stable objects to use under the keyboard and mouse. To test if your keyboard and mouse are at the correct level, check to see if your wrists are flat along with your forearms. The elbows should be directly below the shoulders in a neutral position.

Remember, if you have changed your seat height, you will need to look at your knee angle and foot support. If your seat height is raised, you will need to use a raised surface under your feet, such as a footrest or small box. For a lowered seat, you will need to place your feet further forward, without allowing your hips to slide forward in the seat, e.g., by use of an angled footrest. Ensuring you have continued foot support, and are still getting up and moving around, will help minimize slouching or rounding of the lower back.

Workstations with an adjustable keyboard tray, like one on an adjustable arm or on a height-adjustable work surface, will need the keyboard tray to be adjusted level with your armrests or resting elbow height.

Now that your keyboard surface has been adjusted, the next step is to look at your computer equipment. With the variety of keyboards and mouse devices available, ensuring that these are considered and adjusted for can help alleviate discomfort issues. Devices can be designed to change the users' posture, reduce fatigue, or eliminate keyboard use entirely (voice-based software). We will cover the basics using a standard keyboard and mouse combination and also discuss alternative options and why they work for some but not for others.

## Keyboard

Changing the keyboard allows us to both target the postures they promote while also reducing the buildup of fatigue and strain in the arms and hands. Devices such as a compact keyboard, one without a number pad, are often the first choice for correcting limited work space. In many cases however, compact keyboards end up reducing the key size. This can cause more issues for individuals with wide shoulders or large hands, as it can lead to even greater wrist angles, with similarities seen in individuals who work primarily with a laptop. Individuals who want to address these reaching and leaning postures, but still require the use of a numeric pad, can look into having a compact keyboard with a separate numeric pad, which can be used when needed. Another solution is to use what is called a "left-handed" keyboard, which has a fixed numeric pad on the left side. Computer work, individual physical features, and targeting discomforts should all be considered when looking into alternative keyboards.

The most common approach to target wrist angles is to introduce a split or angled keyboard that provides a fixed or adjustable separation halfway through the keyboard to reduce the need to "tuck" the wrists in. The benefits of these devices can be positive for those who may suffer from wrist related musculoskeletal disorders (MSDs), carpal tunnel being the most common. With that said, they are typically recommended for specific medical issues and require education and fine tuning to find a comfortable position for the user.

As we have talked about the use of physical keyboards, through my work in the past, I have assessed individuals who are unable physically to use a keyboard, whether due to the unfortunate progression of MSD-related injuries or other medical issues. In these cases, the use of a voice-to-text software and microphone setup has allowed them to work at a computer with minimal use of the hands. With the integration of digital assistants, we are seeing an increase in the use of voice-to-text software by the general public. While no longer a specialized product, software that has been made for voice-to-text conversion may provide a more accurate and smooth typing experience compared to the more widely available digital assistants.

As this solution would be catered to an individual. Those who have limitations in their physical ability to use a keyboard, such as due to arthritis, are encouraged to speak with their medical practitioner and employer about voice-to-text options, or consider using it for devices with small input features, such as working off a cellphone.

## Wrist Support

Many computer workstations, both new and old, use a keyboard and/or mouse with a foam or gel wrist support. While these may feel comfortable at the time, there can be long term impacts to wrist health if not used correctly.

How to use wrist supports properly is not intuitive. The concept of a wrist support is simple; provide a soft surface for the wrists and palms to reduce contact pressure on the nerves and blood vessels. When a wrist support is present, it creates an "anchor" point where most or all typing motions are limited to the small muscles of the wrist and palm. This can lead to overuse and repetitive strain injuries, including carpal tunnel syndrome.

The density, material, and size of a wrist rest can all play a part in the amount of strain placed on the wrists. If you decide to use a wrist support, I recommend only using it with the keyboard when you are not typing, such as while reading or thinking. The chair armrests, when adjusted correctly, will provide the forearms and shoulder with support to eliminate the need for a support pad at the wrist(s). While actively typing, "hovering" above the wrist support will promote movement to the larger muscles of the arm that are more resilient.

After we target the keyboard to address wrist and leaning/reaching postures, the next step is to review the mouse device to further target wrist postures.

## Mouse

A standard mouse device tends to be the cause for discomfort in the right forearm and wrist, due to arm positioning. A neutral position for the forearm is with the palm facing "up", with the thumb pointing away from the body. This allows for the two bones in the forearm, the ulna (pinky side) and the radius (thumb side) to be positioned parallel to each other. When we use a standard mouse, however, we are forced to rotate our hands and forearms to a palm down position, which causes the two forearm bones to cross over one another. This can lead to a build-up of tension near the elbow, which can be a contributing factor to developing tennis or golfer's elbow.

Remote work has created a new wrist hazard, especially for workers who use a laptop as their primary computer. What I am referring to, is the use of a touch surface or track pad as the mouse device. This may be convenient for travel or short term use, prolonged use of a track pad on the laptop can lead to wrist, hand, and shoulder discomfort. When we use a track pad, most will end up "hovering" their fingers over the surface while they read. This can lead to tension building up in the top of the hand and forearm as the muscles are constantly active to stop the fingers from moving or "clicking" the cursor. A less obvious, but just as important, impact of using a laptop track pad is the increase reaching distance when typing. By having the mouse below the keyboard, it creates a gap or space that the user must reach over to type, leading to forward leaning postures or overreaching with the arms, causing upper back and shoulder tension to increase. For remote workers who spend the majority of their day on the computer, it is encouraged to use a separate keyboard and mouse to eliminate the hazards of a laptop keyboard and track pad.

Forearm and wrist position can be addressed in two ways: change the position or change the device.

If changing the mouse device is not an option, I would recommend you alternate the hand using the mouse throughout the day. What I mean by this is to start your day with the mouse in your dominant hand and alternate hands and sides throughout the day. Be sure to change your mouse button orientation as well. This is something that I practice daily. By reducing the overuse and strain on one arm and alternating hands, we will help prevent the development of forearm MSDs. There are no time limits on how long to use the mouse in each hand as it varies for each individual. I would encourage you to alternate hands 2 to 3 times per day and use the mouse with the left hand for short periods of time. Slowly building up endurance and accuracy as your comfort, and patience, dictates.

When using the mouse on the left, another common cause of discomfort is addressed, i.e., overreaching with the right arm. With a standard keyboard and mouse combination, assuming the mouse is used with the right hand, we are forced to adopt one of two postures. We either lean on our left elbow to type, or we reach with our right arm and shoulder to use the mouse. By using the mouse with the left hand periodically, we eliminate both of these postures and can sit more upright and centered as the reaching distance of the mouse and keyboard are more balanced to the center of the user.

Changing the mouse device to a vertical mouse will address forearm rotation, as they are designed to be used with a "hand shake" position. This reduces the degree of rotation in the forearm and eliminates movement at the wrist. By decreasing the wrist movement, more shoulder movement is emphasized. This should be taken into consideration for those with shoulder-related injuries. If introducing a vertical mouse, consider keeping a standard mouse nearby to alternate with and gradually increase the time spent using the vertical-style mouse. This will help you adjust to the increased shoulder use and build up endurance. Be aware that if you use this style of device on your right side in combination with a standard keyboard, you will need to be mindful of how much you are leaning and how far you are reaching with the right arm.

When choosing a mouse device, you should also factor in your hand size. Many wireless or "travel" mice are compact in size to be easier to store. However, what this can cause is an increase in hand tension if it is too small. Think about getting "writer's cramp" while writing an essay. This can also afflict the hand if a mouse is too small. The same principle also applies to mouse devices that are too large for the hand. Excessive stretching of the hand due to a large mouse can lead to cramping and muscle fatigue. In the end, where and how you interact with your keyboard and mouse can help to minimize upper-body and arm-related discomforts, staying mindful of your posture and building positive habits to promote variability; taking rest breaks will help you achieve this. Try stretching while you are reading or attending a virtual meeting. Use rest periods to help alleviate tension and tightness so that you can work happier at your desk.

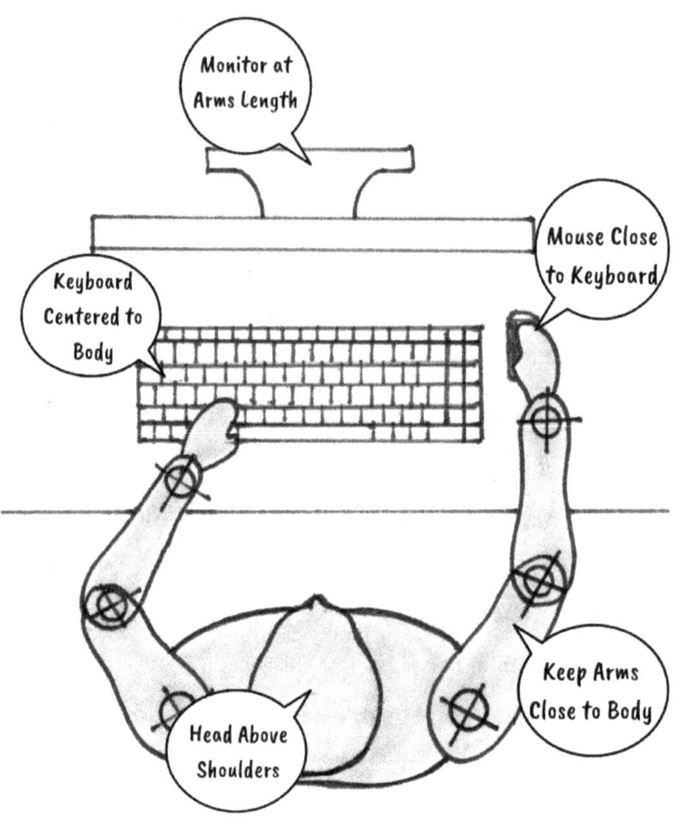


**Figure 3.2**: Keyboard and Mouse Quick Reference

# Section 4: Screens

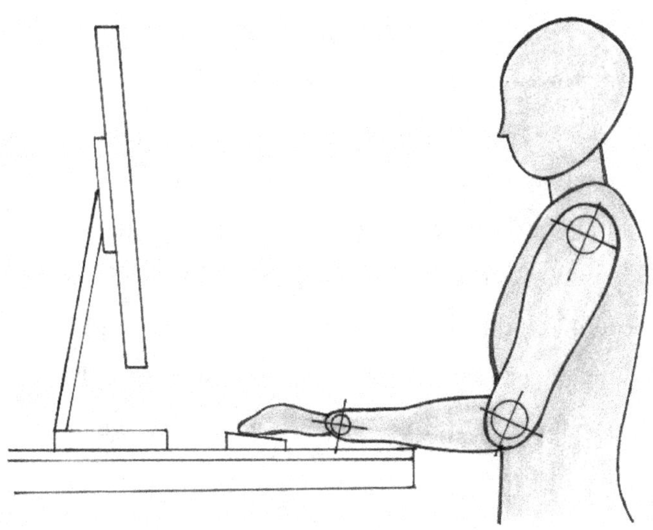

**Figure 4.1**: Screens

The multiple screens that we stare at on a daily basis are one of the main contributors to neck and shoulder discomfort, especially when they are poorly adjusted. With the increase in digital work, many standard office workstations are also outfitted with two monitors. The positioning of these screens can affect viewing height, angle, and eye fatigue. Sitting for too long at a computer screen or on the phone in a poor position, or working on a laptop, are common contributors to discomfort and can lead to tension headaches. When we consider the use of computer screens, cellphones, laptops, and/or tablets, a great deal of time is spent on screens, which highlights the importance of ensuring they are properly positioned. Making a small height change of 1 inch or 2.5 cm can be a great relief to the muscles in the neck.

This section will cover the basics of adjusting single and dual screen monitor setups, positioning of a laptop as the primary or secondary monitor, and proper positioning for a tablet or cellphone. We will also cover tips to help individuals wearing different corrective lenses to ensure they position their screen at the appropriate height.

## External Monitors

The first adjustment you want to make is to have the height set to where your eyes align with the top ⅓ of the screen when looking forward. A good marker is to have your eyes lined up with the bottom of the toolbar in a Word document. This allows viewing of the screen to be primarily by eye movement with minimal neck movement. If your screen is too high you should adjust the monitor stand, lower the surface the screen is on, or raise your chair. Keep in mind that if you raise your chair, you will need to use or adjust your foot support, as discussed in Section 3, to prevent lower limb discomfort. If your screen is too low, try raising the screen by adjusting the built-in stand or, if it does not have adjustability, place a couple of books underneath your monitor. For those who want a wider range of adjustability, whether for multiple users or adjustability based on the work, a single/dual screen monitor arm setup will allow for a much greater range of both height, angle, distance between monitors, and viewing distance. When looking for a monitor arm setup, you want to make sure it can be securely mounted to your desk surface to prevent it from falling.

Especially with an aging workforce, we must consider the differences in corrective lenses as it will affect viewing height and angle. For individuals who wear bifocal or progressive glasses, where the lower half of the glasses is for reading, you want your eyes to line up with the top of the screen when looking forwards. This will prevent you from having to tilt the head up when reading.

## Laptop Screen

The monitor height should also be reflected in laptop screen use, albeit with a couple of additional changes. Since most laptop screens cannot be separated from the laptop body, it is strongly encouraged to place the laptop on a raised surface and use an external keyboard and mouse. This will give you more adjustability to set up the laptop screen to a comfortable height without forcing improper hand and shoulder posture by using the laptop keyboard and trackpad. I find using a stack of paper (typically 2 inches or 5 cm high) or textbooks to be effective risers for a laptop.

## Distance and Positioning

How far away you place your screen(s) will play a key role in back, neck, and arm posture. A general rule of thumb is to have your monitors positioned an arm's length away. This allows for the information on the screen to be at a comfortable reading distance to prevent leaning forward or slouching. If your work involves highly detailed documents or images, it may be beneficial to zoom the file window or bring the screen(s) closer. Just be sure to take more visual breaks when working closer to the monitor to minimize the buildup of eye strain.

Adjusting your monitor angle will also help to minimize the head from tilting forward leaning when reading. For most individuals, you want to adjust your monitors with a slight tilt backwards (e.g., a 95° angle). The reason why we angle our screens can be best described with the analogy of chopping wood. When chopping wood, you would swing an axe from above the head, downwards onto a log. As the axe moves down, the blade does not move in a straight line, it follows an arc or curve. This is similar to how our viewing distance changes as our eyes look down the monitor. When you are reading something on the monitor and your eyes are moving downwards, the screen should be tilted slightly back to maintain the same viewing distance, or trying to more closely match the viewing "arc". This will help reduce eye strain, due to constant refocusing, as well as reducing the habit of leaning forwards.

If you are fortunate to have two monitors at your workstation, you want to consider the amount of time spent on each screen when adjusting their position. If you spend the majority of your time working on one over the other, then you should position that screen to be more directly in front to reduce turning of the neck. If time spent between the two screens is about equal, then you will want the touching edges of the screens centered on you.

The office environment will also play a role in monitor positioning, especially when lighting can affect visibility. Monitors should be placed in a location that is perpendicular to a window, to minimize glare on the screen, and offset from overhead lighting to reduce glare. This will also help reduce eye strain from reflected sunlight, or from light shining directly in your face.

## Minimizing Eye Strain

Like taking a physical break from sitting at your desk, you should also take a visual break from staring at your monitor(s). Some of the muscles in the eyes are used to help focus on close objects, and some are used for distance. If we spend too much time focused at the same distance, these eye muscles become fatigued which can lead to difficulty reading and blurry vision. At least once every hour you should look away from the screen and focus on something distant. This could be looking at something outside or across the room. Another thing to remember is to blink. Yes, blinking is reduced when working on a screen due to blue light stimulating our brains. This can lead to drying out of the surface of our eyes resulting in itchiness and redness. By moving your eyes around, and taking breaks from the computer, we can ensure that we blink and keep our eyes well hydrated. A quick way to help relax strained eye muscles, while also rehydrating our eyes, is to close the eyes and place the warm palms of our hands over them. The heat from the palm will warm up and relax the eye muscles while the closed eyelid allows the surface of our eyes to rehydrate.

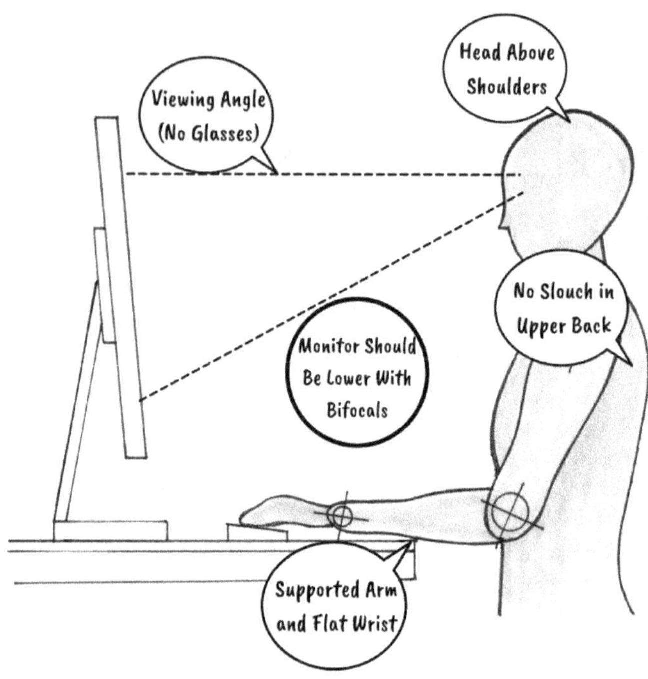


**Figure 4.2**: Screens Quick Reference

# Section 5: Desk Surface

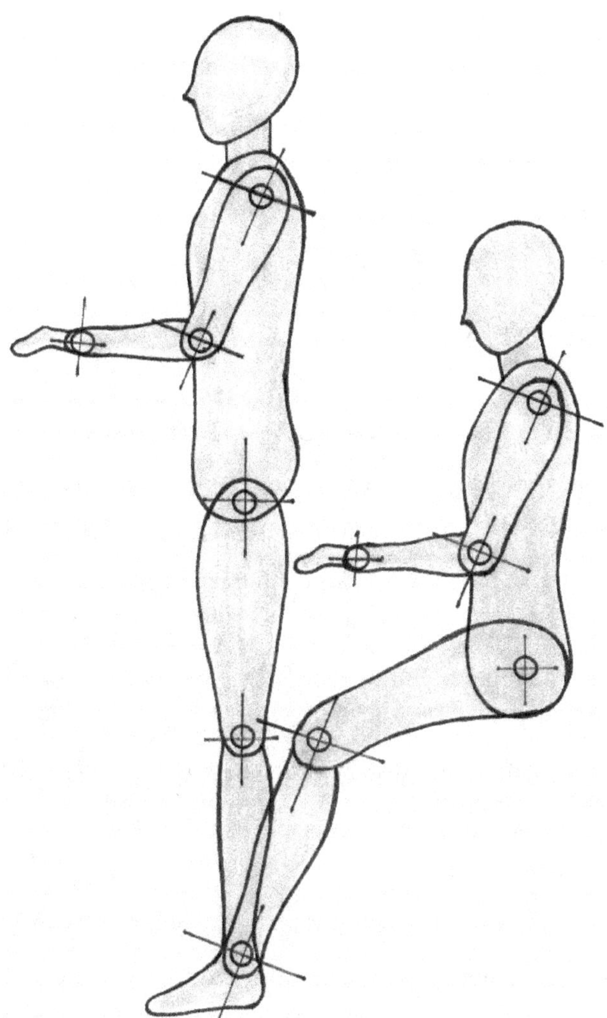

**Figure 5.1**: Desk Surface

The desk is central to the computer setup and provides space for our office materials, computers, and peripherals. By efficiently placing documents and other objects around ourselves, we can minimize leaning and excessive reaching postures. This section will provide a discussion on the variety in work surfaces, tips on how to achieve a comfortable desk height regardless of what you are using, and a discussion on sit/stand workstations.

## The Desk

There are a few common features we want to consider when choosing a desk. You want to find a desk that you can comfortably sit at, have it located in a dedicated location, and that has enough space for your computer equipment and peripherals. This could be a desk, a table, or a kitchen island. I have used both a desk and dining table for my home office setups and the trick is to adjust your setup to accommodate the work surface. The difficulty in using something like the dining table is that you are constantly moving your "office" to accommodate meals, family, or a significant other also using it as an office. There is also limited ability to "adjust" it for the computer equipment. By having a dedicated workstation, we are able to set things up properly the first time without having to worry about how to make it easier to move or disassemble.

Work surfaces, such as dining tables, pose a challenge in achieving that "custom" fit for the keyboard and mouse as the height of the equipment is dependent on the table height. While this may be at the correct height for some, the vast majority of individuals will find that a desk or table is too high for their keyboard and mouse. Over time, this can lead to an increase in upper back and arm discomfort. To ensure the equipment is adjusted to the right height, without taking a saw to the table legs (which may upset your significant other), you should raise your seated height by raising the chair height or by sitting on a cushion.

## Sit/Stand Desk

To improve the flexibility of postures at the workstation, we have seen the rise in popularity of height-adjustable workstations, which we will refer to as sit/stand desks. The term sit/stand desk refers to either a free standing desk with a height adjustable base, or equipment used on a fixed surface that can raise the computer for use while standing. This equipment allows the user to adjust the height of their computer and equipment for use while seated or standing, depending on their preference, and provides the adjustability to accommodate a wider range of individual heights.

If you are considering purchasing, or are using and sit/stand desk, I will highlight some of the pros and cons of using these devices and how to adjust and use them correctly. I would not recommend a sit/stand desk for everyone as its use and benefits are highly dependent on the person and their situation. Part of this section will cover alternative ways of achieving posture variation without the need for a sit/stand desk or drastic changes to the workstation.

Focused on helping those with lower back discomfort, sit/stand desks work by reducing the static sitting posture, a primary cause of discomfort for many, and allow the user to vary their posture throughout the day. With increasing popularity, especially in North America, it is seen as a cost-effective and proactive way to reduce discomfort and improve employee morale and wellbeing. The implementation of sit/stand desks, however, has shown conflicting results in recent research, where some indicate little to no impact on reducing lower back discomfort and others indicating positive results. A key factor in the success of a sit/stand solution is the training involved in its implementation and use.

To determine whether a sit/stand desk may be appropriate for you, you should consider the pros and cons and their impact on you.

*The pros of using a sit/stand desk can include:*

1. It allows for a high amount of posture variability throughout the day.

2. It promotes a more "neutral" posture in the lower back and hips when standing by reducing rounding and slouching.

3. It promotes more blood flow by reducing contact pressure on the legs and increasing movement.

4. It prevents leaning at the shoulders or hips for long periods.

*The cons of using a sit/stand desk can include:*

1. It increases pressure on the feet, knees, and hips, especially when standing on hard surfaces.

2. It lacks shoulder/arm support which puts pressure on wrists and increases shoulder and back tension.

3. It is higher cost and more space dependent.

4. It is dependent on proper education/training in use for it to be effective.

When using a sit/stand desk, you need to understand that adjusting your body to the change will take time and should not be rushed. Muscle tension, ongoing injuries and recovery, and footwear will all have an effect on how well your body adjusts to the equipment.

Especially for new users, you will need to start off slow with short durations of standing followed by walking or sitting to prevent the build-up of discomfort while your body adjusts. A good rule of thumb to follow is to start with 10 minutes of standing followed by 50 minutes of sitting. As your body adapts to standing more often, you can increase the standing time. While a timer may be useful to remind us to change position, we want to use posture indicators that you can watch out for that indicate you have been standing for too long. These can include; leaning on the left or right hip, tightness in the back and hips, sore or swelling feet, locking or hyperextending the knees, upper body slouching, and leaning on the desk/keyboard surface.

When using a sit/stand desk, the principles regarding adjusting it for monitor and keyboard height are different to those when working in a primarily seated position. With some minor adjustments to what was covered earlier in this book, we can ensure they are adjusted correctly. The height of your monitor(s) and keyboard/mouse will continue to be based on eye level and elbow heights respectively. However, since there is no arm support from a chair while standing, and the back is in a more upright position, the distance between the monitor and keyboard heights will be greater when standing. To adjust for this, you should first adjust the keyboard surface to the standing elbow height, and then raise the monitor to the correct viewing height. Don't forget to reset these adjustments when moving back to a seated posture.

There are three additional items I would encourage you to consider while using a sit/stand desk. The first is a pair of comfortable shoes. Shoes that fit well, provide arch support, and have adequate cushioning can reduce pressure on the feet, especially if you are standing on a hard surface for prolonged periods of time. Secondly, consider looking into a footrest or small stool underneath the desk. By alternating one of your feet on the stool when standing, similar to what you would find at a bar/pub counter, it will reduce pressure on the hip and leg joints (this method is commonly used in retail by cashiers). The third and final item is a good quality anti-fatigue mat with slip-resistant surfacing. This will provide additional cushioning when standing to reduce contact stress on the feet by better distributing the body weight. Whether you use a sit/stand desk or the kitchen table, spending a bit of time assessing and adjusting your desk surface can make a world of difference on your comfort and physical health.

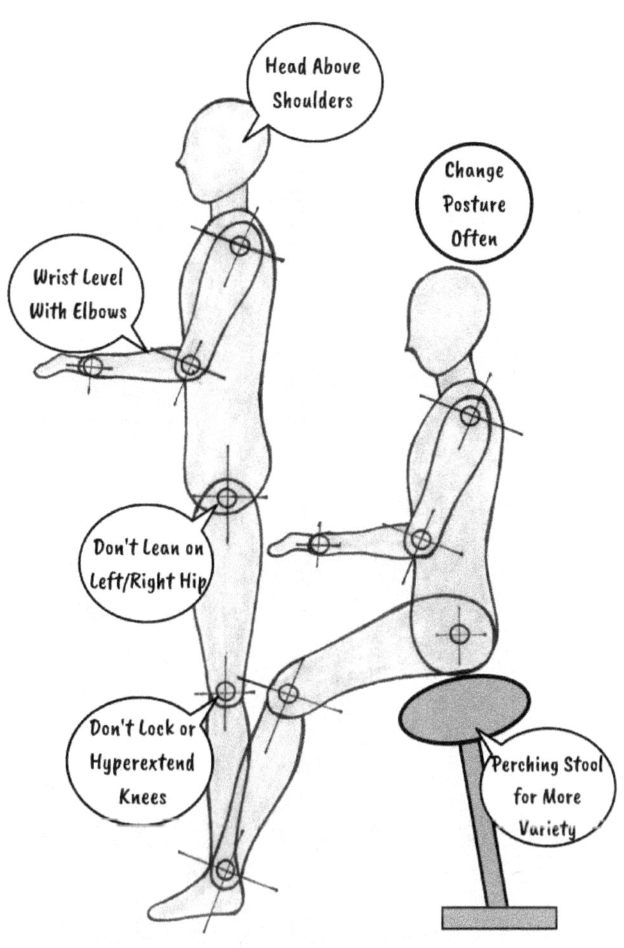



**Figure 5.2**: Desk Surface Quick Reference

# Section 6: Peripherals

With the changes in our office environments, we need to include a brief discussion on peripherals used on a daily basis. For this section, we will focus on printed materials, desk lights, and phones as these are the most common peripherals found in offices.

## Documents

Depending on your work, you may or may not use printed materials. With the increase in digital documentation, both for environmental and organization benefits, more of our reference materials are accessed on the computer. There are still some that, like me, will have several printed documents that are referenced throughout the day. Whether it's a report, textbook, or an engineered drawing, having a comfortable position for these printed documents will help minimize neck strain and leaning. For those who spend a large part of their day working with printed materials, I would encourage you to purchase a 2 page document holder. This will allow for documents to be placed at a more upright position, reducing the forwards head tilt, and even decreasing leaning on the left or right shoulder. Alternatively, a quick and easy fix is by placing your printed material on an empty 3-ring binder. The binder will act as a "wedge" to angle the documents, much like a document holder, but has the added benefit of being able to support a larger amount of weight, such as from a heavy textbook.

## Task Lights

Task or desk lights are a relatively standard item in North American offices, whether it is sitting directly on the desk or attached underneath a shelf. The placement and use of task lighting can provide an office with a more balanced lighting environment, helping to reduce eye strain. When using a task light in the office, ideally one with adjustable brightness, the location of the light is important depending on what you are doing. The first use of a task light, as the name suggests, is to provide additional light on a specific item, such as a book or reference document. This will aid in visual comfort and reducing eye strain when reading or reviewing detailed information by providing a more comfortable light level.

When choosing a location for office lighting, you want to make sure that it is not placed behind your monitors or behind you. Lighting behind the monitors can cause an imbalance where the screen appears dimmer, making it harder for the eyes to focus. Lighting directly behind you will create a glare on the monitor, making it difficult to read what is on the screen. The best location for office lighting is above and slightly to the side, or to the left/right of your monitors, depending on where you place your cellphone or hard copy materials.

Task lighting can also be used when working in a dimly lit office, or when natural/overhead lighting is lacking, to supplement the lighting environment. This can also be done depending on the time of day. For example, if you have an office that is primarily supplied by natural light, such as from a window, task lighting may be used earlier and/or later in the day to supplement sunrise and sunset light levels. Enclosed offices with little or no natural light, and rely on fluorescent lighting, can use a task light to provide a more comfortable yellowish or "natural" light, mimicking sunlight. Since our eyes are naturally adjusted to the yellow light, it reduces the strain "white" light, produced by most artificial lighting, can cause on the eyes.

There are specialized task lighting, such as "D Lights" available on the market to closely simulate natural sunlight and are typically used for individuals suffering from Seasonal Affective Disorder (SAD). As this item is more specific to the individual, I would strongly encourage you to seek the advice from your medical practitioner to understand if it would be the right option for you.

In most cases, a dimmable LED task light is ideal for offices as it allows the user to customize the light levels while also being more energy efficient.

## Phone Use

Desk phones and cellphones, and how they are used, play a key role in today's office environment. With the increased use of these devices, making sure you have the proper setup can make the work day easier and pain-free. If your job requires frequent phone use, make sure to place it within arm's reach. This will help reduce leaning and overreaching which can prevent pressure and strain from building up on your hips and shoulders.

Placing your phone on the same side as your dominant hand can also reduce shoulder and back discomfort. The reason for this is that, out of habit, most individuals will answer their phone by picking it up with the dominant hand first, regardless of what side of the body it is on. By placing the phone on the dominant side, you are no longer reaching across the body and twisting the spine.

As businesses continue to increase their reliance on cellphones, there has been a subsequent increase in neck related injuries, such as "text neck". The placement of cellphone or tablet screens can be used to minimize or prevent the development of such injuries. Raising your tablet or cellphone screen while using it can decrease the forward tilting of the head, taking pressure off the neck joints and muscles. If you are using a tablet or cellphone as the primary device, a really easy tip for raising the screen while seated is by placing something under the elbows, such as a pillow, or underneath the device. This will prop the device higher, improving neck posture, as we want to treat it like a monitor and have it as close to a comfortable viewing height as we can. It is very important while using the phone, not just in the office but at any time, that you should avoid the bad posture of cradling or holding the phone between your head and shoulder. This posture creates a large amount of strain on the neck muscles and uneven pressure on the cervical spine/neck. While there are devices, such as cushions or attachments, used on desk phones to increase the phone handset size, it still promotes the same posture, albeit to a lesser degree. If you are frequently answering the phone or attending long conference calls/meetings, I would strongly encourage using a hands-free headset, either with earbuds, Bluetooth headphones, or a traditional call center style headset. This will free up your hands to use the computer or reference printed documents while also eliminating the strain on the neck and shoulder.

# Section 7: Closing Notes

 Whether you are new to the office environment, or have been working in one for most of your life, I hope the information provided throughout this book has taught you to understand what postures work best for you.

With the awareness and knowledge to assess and correct the ergonomic hazards at your workstation, you will have a pain-free office and a happier life. One of the foundations to maintaining a healthy and pain-free office is frequent movement throughout the day. By combining the adjustments you have made to your office, with frequent movement, you too can live and work healthier.

By no means are the adjustments that you have made today the "final setup" and nothing should be glued in place. What you have learned is the ability to adapt any workstation to fit you, making you more versatile and efficient.

I wish you the best of luck in your working lives and hope you enjoy a pain-free life outside the office.

Looking for more ways to connect? Check out my website for more information and links to my social media accounts.

www.informedsafety.com

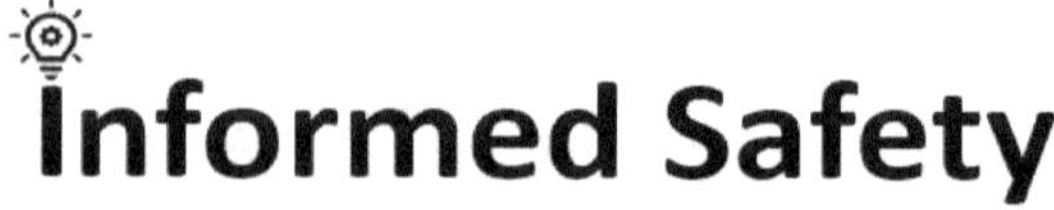

www.ingramcontent.com/pod-product-compliance
Lightning Source LLC
Chambersburg PA
CBHW070043260726
48658CB00002B/715